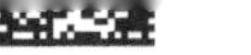

Bond mason

THE 5 SECRET ON HOW TO LOSE WEIGHT AND PLAN FOR A FLAT BELLY

Introduction

Losing Weight with an Algorithm that
Actually Works + Diet Tips

Losing weight is not easy. It takes a lot of
time, effort, and dedication. But what if
you could lose weight with an algorithm
that actually works? And even better,
what if you could lose weight while eating
the foods you love?

This article is all about how to lose weight
with an algorithm that actually works and
diet tips to get started.

chapter 1

THE BENEFITS OF HEALTHY DIET PLAN

A healthy diet plan can have a significant impact on your life. It can help you to lose weight, maintain a healthy lifestyle and avoid diseases.

There are many benefits of a healthy diet plan, such as:

- Weight Loss

- Disease Prevention

- A Healthy Lifestyle

A healthy diet plan is essential for a healthy lifestyle. A diet plan can be as simple as following a few guidelines or it can be more complex. The benefits of following a healthy diet plan are:

- Reduces the risk of chronic diseases - Improves mental health - Promotes weight loss or weight maintenance - Provides emotional support - Promotes better sleep - Improves physical activity levels

A healthy diet plan is essential for a healthy lifestyle. A diet plan can be as simple as following a few guidelines or it can be more complex. The benefits of following a healthy diet plan are:

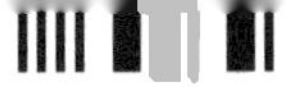

- Reduces the risk of chronic diseases - Improves mental health - Promotes weight loss or weight maintenance - Provides emotional support - Promotes better sleep - Improves physical activity

chapter 2

WHAT TO EAT ON A HEALTHY DIET PLAN

If you are looking for a healthy diet plan, there are plenty of options out there. The best one for you will depend on your personal preferences and the lifestyle that you lead.

There are many reasons why people choose to eat a healthy diet, but they usually fall into two camps: those who want to lose weight or those who want to maintain their weight.

The first step in creating a healthy diet plan is figuring out what your goals are. Once you know that, it becomes much easier to create a plan that will help you achieve them.

—

The most important part of a healthy diet plan is to eat a variety of foods. It is important to eat vegetables, fruits, whole grains, and protein sources.

People should try to avoid sugar-sweetened beverages and food items that contain high amounts of sugar. They should also try to avoid processed meats such as bacon and sausage.

It is important to start with what you are going to eat. This will be the foundation for your diet plan. You should eat a variety of foods that are healthy and nutritious.

It is recommended to eat something from each of these five food groups: vegetables, fruits, whole grains, lean protein, and dairy products.

If you want to lose weight or maintain your weight, it is important to limit the amount of calories you consume each day. It is recommended that women who are sedentary

should have 1,200 calories per day and men who are sedentary should have 1,500 calories per day.

chapter 3

What You Get to Eat on a Healthy Diet that Will Help You Lose Weight

A healthy diet is essential to weight loss. Studies show that even if you are not eating a lot, if your diet is not healthy, you will not lose weight.

A healthy diet consists of vegetables, fruits, whole grains, lean proteins and low-fat dairy products. These foods are high in fiber and nutrients that keep you feeling full for longer periods of time. This means that you will have less cravings for unhealthy food and will be able to maintain a healthier weight.

chapter 4

We'll have warm ajwain water.

you should simply warm

 two teaspoons of ajwain in water

for a few minutes and have its

bicep void stomach

continuing   towards   our
morning meal for

which i'll give both of you to
three choices

initial one will be indian pizza
now

the recipe is really simple it is
referenced

hair so the thing I'm doing
here is in a

bowl i'll add around six

teaspoon of suji and to this
i'll be

adding again greek yogurt
you can utilize

hunger additionally or you
can utilize typical curd

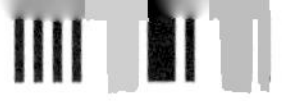

additionally and to this i'll
add red chime

peppers   yellow   chime
peppers green

capsicum smashing out pink
himalayan

salt dark pepper powder and
afterward i'll

be including a water to mix
everything

up you can shape it into a
decent glue

until you see this consistency
now in a

container i'll add just

one teaspoon of olive oil

what's more, i'll toast my
bread cut up

subsequent to toasting it

i'll apply the player on this side

also, spreading everything well now once it is

all spreaded well

flip it over don't stress the blend

won't adhere to the dish as a
result of

curd let it toast appropriately
and afterward you

see this wonderful

indian pizza really simple
very yummy to

plan and trust me so bright
that

the   children   will   likewise
adore having this you

might actually add parmesan
cheddar or sprinkle

some nourishing yeast over it
for good

vitamin b12 and b6

what's   more,   for   a   messy
surface too you can

have up to two sound indian
pizzas

while you're having this for
your

dinner and appreciate it well
alongside this

you can have tear espresso
according to your own

inclination yet with no sugar
you can

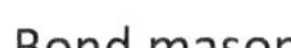

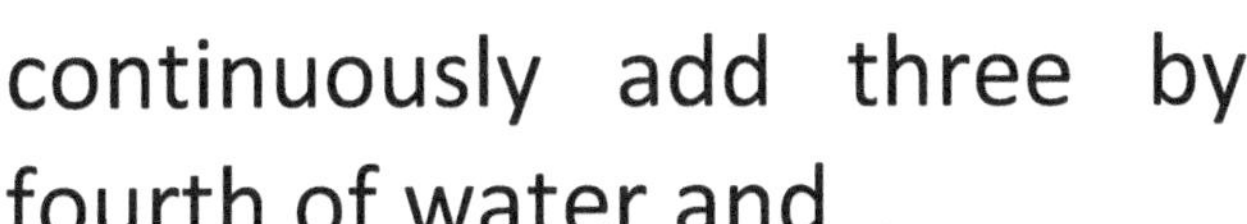

continuously add three by
fourth of water and

one by fourth of milk in the
tea or

espresso to make it more

weight   reduction   situated
subsequent choice for

your morning meal will be
apple nut

margarine smoothie now the
recipe for apple

peanut butter smoothie is
hair frozen

banana one frozen apple
peanut butter it

is effectively accessible on
the lookout

you can get it on the web or
an apple one

frozen banana you can freeze
it

short-term and some almond
milk now you

can take a standard milk
likewise on the off chance
that you

like as such however I utilize
just almond

milk one tablespoon of
peanut butter now

you should simply in a
blender take

this large number of fixings
put it in the

blender and mix it for
somewhere around two

minutes   presently   i'm
utilizing the normal

blender   with   new   apple
some finely

hacked nuts here i'm utilizing

almond   and   pecans   and
alongside that I

add some

newly   pre-arranged   home
granola or you can

likewise add muesli to this it
gives a very

tasty crunchy flavor to the
pleasant

cream third choice for your
paunch fat

misfortune breakfast will be

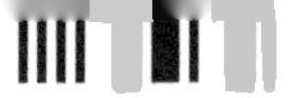

for all the workplace
attendees and who need to

convey their morning meal
really effectively oats

clearly in a portion of some
milk and half

cup of water added you
could in fact add parts

what's more, heaps of
organic product to this also
to

make it more full

presently   we   should
continue towards an early in
the day

nibble for which i'll be giving
you

basic   one   choice   very
compelling for

losing all the paunch fat
region and as

well as to give your body
great

cell reinforcement levels too
it very well may be

either green tea or matcha
tea now one

cup of matcha tea is
equivalent to 10 cups of

green   tea   the   cell
reinforcement level in that

specific one cup of matcha
tea will be

a lot higher than some other
superfood purchase

the best matcha tea it's

given in the portrayal box
beneath you

can proceed to look at it
continuing

towards our lunch and one
hour prior

our lunch we'll have apple
juice vinegar

in tepid water

today i'll present you all with

quite possibly of the best

apple   juice   vinegars   the
market these

days   that   is   new   spices
natural apple

juice vinegar

the most awesome aspect of
this specific

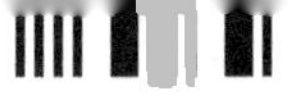

apple juice vinegar is it is crude and

natural it is produced using himalayan apples

furthermore, it's naturally ensured 100 unadulterated

furthermore, regular mother protein which is a stomach

cordial microbes is vital when

taken   with   apple   juice
vinegar

it's no additives and the key

benefits   for   apple   juice
vinegar is it

helps in weight reduction it
brings down your

glucose levels and works on
your

processing without any problem

consumes stomach fat rapidly attempt it for

multi week and you'll see the outcomes

yourself

you should simply add two teaspoons

of apple juice vinegar

in a glass and heated water to this

blend it well and taste it.

chapter 5

One hour before your lunch

To   obtain   the   most   ideal outcomes for

this beverage

purchase   new   spices   natural apple juice

vinegar the connection is given in the

depiction box beneath you can proceed to purchase

it and look at it yourself have it
for

multi week and you'll see the
outcomes

yourself

what's more, presently we
should continue towards our
lunch

choices lunch choices i'll be
giving you

first being veggie kitchen now the

recipe for veggie kitchen

have it alongside curd and salad and

you'll   appreciate   having   it subsequent choice

will be you can have either mushroom or

paneer sabzi with a plate of
mixed greens this is going

to be a no cup or low carb

lunch choices for every one of
the individuals who can have

it and have egg curry assuming
that you like having

eggs for your lunch

cultivating towards our third
choice for

lunch will be oats with natural products

presently the recipe for my oats with

natural products or a fast cereal recipe here is

the total recipe it's really simple to

plan add more

milk or water to this and set it
up in

a fluid structure on the off
chance that you could do
without it to

be adequately strong

have it alongside endlessly loads
of

newly   organic   products
accessible that is papaya

banana   mango apple   berries whatever is

accessible with you and have it for your

lunch you continue towards our

mid-night nibble for which i'll be

giving you one choice which will be

dark espresso with added lemon juice to

it functions as a very fat terminator attempt it

yourself for two days and you'll see

your stomach fat diminishing to an incredible

degree you should simply get ready

dark espresso and add

a portion of a lemon press to it
and have it

warm

continuing towards our

supper for which i'll be giving
you

three choices the first will be

pineapple smoothie pineapple is
a

regular fat shaper and certainly will

lessen your tummy fat to a more noteworthy

degree you should simply just

mix

one cup of pineapple a portion of a banana

some curd or yogurt or milk according to your

own decision or you could add water as

well for the consistency clean everything

also, have it sit by taste for your supper

subsequent choice will be sound almond

milk haldi or turmeric is again an incredible

cell   reinforcement   level   and
calming

too so make a point to add new

desi haldi for this and ready in

almond   milk   just   third   choice
will be

for every one of the people who
like to have servings of mixed
greens

for their supper which will be
paneer

salad or soya salad or egg salad
egg

whites just and not the yolk part

paneer

or then again soya you can
utilize 70 grams of it and

incorporate endlessly heaps of
salad to this

cucumber tomato lettuce onion
whatever

is uncommonly accessible with
you add it

to it no salt to the serving of
mixed greens since it's

just in a crude structure won't
have crude

salt in any structure

make the dressing with concrete
or

yogurt

lemon juice dark pepper powder
oregano

bean stew chips

appreciate having the serving of
mixed greens for your supper

continuing   towards   our   sleep
time drink

which will be really significant for

this diet plan which will be jeera water

jeera once more

assists you with decreasing your water regard for

a three oil two teaspoons of jeera in

one entire glass of water

allow it to stew for something
like two minutes

also, have it sit by taste prior to
going to

bed you love having this sleep
time bring

as you see the outcomes
yourself.